Massage Therapy Insights:
What You Need To Know

Massage Therapy Insights: What You Need To Know

Practical Applications from Hands-on Experience

HEIDI J. FAGLEY

iUniverse, Inc.
New York Lincoln Shanghai

Massage Therapy Insights: What You Need To Know
Practical Applications from Hands-on Experience

iUniverse books may be ordered through booksellers or by contacting:

iUniverse
2021 Pine Lake Road, Suite 100
Lincoln, NE 68512
www.iuniverse.com
1-800-Authors (1-800-288-4677)

ISBN: 978-0-595-45134-0 (pbk)
ISBN: 978-0-595-89446-8 (ebk)

Printed in the United States of America

This book is dedicated to everyone who touches the lives of others as a massage therapist. May you receive as much as you give.

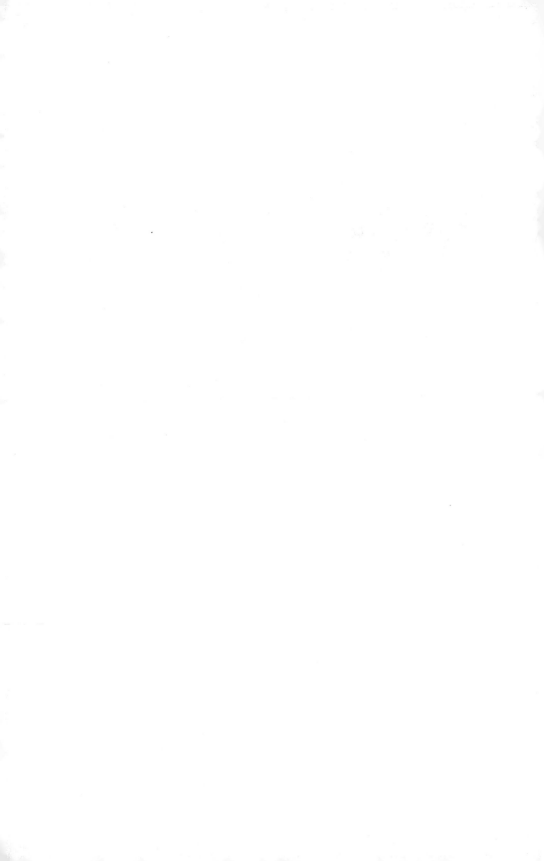

"We make a Living by what we get, but we make a Life by what we give."

—Winston Churchill

INTRODUCTION

The purpose of this book is to limit some of the surprises and "What-do-I-do-now?" situations you may encounter during your career as a massage therapist, because it is guaranteed that you *will* experience some very unusual circumstances with your clients from time to time. The better prepared you are, the more professional you will appear than if you get "caught off guard."

First and foremost: being polite and taking the feelings of your clients into consideration is of the utmost importance. When something is embarrassing for them, you will want to minimize their discomfort about it–whatever it is. Granted, certain things will be quite funny, or difficult, or downright annoying. But whatever it is, you will need to be able to control your reactions. In a field such as ours the phrase "Forewarned is Forearmed" can be one of your best allies!

This book will shed some light on some of the probabilities awaiting you and offer suggestions and remedies to smooth your way. The subjects covered have been chosen from actual personal experiences that occurred during my years of practicing massage. You will be introduced to all types of personalities, moods, sizes, and shapes. It was quite an education going to work each day not knowing what new adventures I would find waiting for me on the table. They brought me challenges, joy and laughter–and everything in between. I'm hoping my Moments to Remember will provide you with insights about how you may decide to handle some strange, awkward, and uncomfortable situations and circumstances that can–and probably will–present themselves quite unexpectedly!

Use these golden rules for greater success in your career:

- Treat each person and each situation with kindness.

- Take the time to listen to your clients and to learn their specific needs and concerns.

- The more you treat each person as a unique individual, the more satisfying and fulfilling your experiences as a massage therapist will be.

- Last but not least, remember your clients are naked and that means they're vulnerable. Treat them with the respect you would wish for yourself in such a situation.

PREFACE

Since graduating from massage therapy school in 1991 I have had the opportunity to work with thousands of interesting and fascinating individuals. Each person I had the privilege of spending time with taught me something valuable about humanity in general. The differences in personalities, body types, and conditions greatly expanded my awareness and understanding of anatomy, physiology, and sociology in reality.

Working in all types of environments and eventually teaching massage, I was often asked about my experiences. "What's the strangest/grossest/weirdest thing that has ever happened?" Or, "Has 'this' or 'that' ever happened?" And, "How did you handle it?" The answers to those many questions are what comprise this book. Another reason for sharing my experiences in this way is because I honestly wish I would have had something like this book to use as a reference. Hearing that I wasn't "alone" in facing all the unknowns awaiting me and having the advice to help prepare me for different types of experiences would have been a real comfort! I hope you will find it so.

I greatly believe in massage therapy and the benefits it provides the body/mind/spirit. My career has provided me with an education about the human race in ways no other career could have given me. If you have picked up this book because you are in school to become a massage therapist, are thinking of becoming a massage therapist, or for whatever the reason you are reading these words, please understand that, although these pages are filled with situations and circumstances that are not necessarily showing the best aspects massage has to offer, each experience helped me grow into a more empathetic, intuitive, and grateful individual. Working in this field has been a privilege–one that I have honored and taken seriously. After all is said and done, the majority of people you massage during your career will be a delight. They will love how you make them feel and will praise you unconditionally. Referrals are made, and clients become regulars you see and get to know well over the years.

Massage therapists have the opportunity to touch people's lives in ways you may never comprehend, because no one can possibly fathom the impact non-judgmental acceptance and simple kindness can make in any one life. A client once said to me as the massage was ending, "That was the nicest thing anyone has ever done for me." I carry those words with me; they touched my whole being. It's a great career when, daily, people are telling you how great they feel and how wonderful you are! What is important is to make sure you do not judge who you are and/or the mood you'll be in if someone does *not* comment on how extraordinary you are! Be confident and stay humble no matter what they say.

DISCLAIMER

My heartfelt appreciation is extended to all the clients who have given me the experiences I have used in this book as a reference for others. I have the deepest respect and gratitude for each person who came to my table and provided me with the opportunity to understand more about tolerance, sensitivity, acceptance, and so much more.

This book has been written with the greatest of care to avoid offensiveness to any one of my clients. My sole purpose in sharing the experiences in this book is to provide increased awareness in a positive and instructional way to those who enter the field of massage therapy.

ACKNOWLEDGEMENTS

Chandler, for listening and being my trusted confidant. Thank you for suggesting I take my career experiences and turn them into a book so others can learn from them. You have supported me in following my dreams, while teaching me how to explore the deeper part of what is most important to me.

Mom, I couldn't have done this without you! Editing every word and being there for me so willingly and unconditionally in every way through every process of this endeavor and throughout my life has been a gift.

Dad, you are such a steadfast grounding force for me. Teaching me to take something positive from every person and experience I encounter in life has been priceless.

My sister, Jill, for your true sisterhood. I am grateful for your love.

My brother-in-law, Bill, for his sore shoulders so I always have someone to work on!

And my nephews, Skylar and Garrett–you are both equally and individually the lights of my life.

My sincere appreciation to everyone who has believed in me and supported my creative spirit.

Thank you to each person who has carried my table for me!!!

A deep gratitude to every client who has been a part of my career. I thank you for providing me with the opportunity to learn as much about humankind as I have about the human body. Each of you has changed my life and taught me things in ways I otherwise may never have learned.

CONTENTS

SECTION I

CLOTHING AND TABLE MANNERS
Caution: Personalities, Egos, And Issues Involved Here!

The bottom line here is to *Be Specific*. And I do mean explain *exactly* what the client's role is in this two-person endeavor that is about to occur! Having asked clients if they had received massages previously, many gave me an affirmative reply such as, "All the time." My mistake (initially) was in assuming they understood how to prepare themselves when I left the room after our pre-massage chat. However, to cite a few instances:

- One woman kept her underwear and bra on.
- One woman kept her clothes on and got under the sheets.
- One man took off the proper clothing but got under *all* the sheets and blankets and was lying directly on the surface of the massage table.
- One man didn't take his clothes off and was lying directly on the table *over* the sheets and blanket.
- One man took *everything* off and was lying on *top* of the sheets and blanket!

Obviously I quickly learned how to adapt my pre-massage chat to include such situations! (I could have made good use of this book!)

There are many times when especially first-time massage clients will feel a bit self-conscious and want to keep as much of their clothing on as possible. To put your clients at ease, explain the draping procedure you use during the massage and assure them you will never see anything inappropriate. Tell men and women alike they may choose to keep their underwear on if they would be more comfortable, but everything else will need to be removed to allow you to work on the back, neck, and other areas where clothing would be a hindrance. If they become regular clients, they will undoubtedly realize the benefit to them and the convenience to you in removing all their clothing.

Explain to women they can keep their bra on, but when they are lying on their tummy, you will unhook the bra to better access the muscles in the back *if they are comfortable with that*. Most of the time, once you begin the massage and they understand how the whole experience works and what to expect, they will relax. When a woman is breast-feeding, she may choose to keep her bra on. Explain that will be fine. You may want to ask her if moving her bra straps down to work on her shoulders and unhooking her bra to work on her back would be okay. More times than not this will be fine with them, but if not, work as she wishes. I've done it both ways.

Comments you might add beyond the usual explanations and instructions will depend on the more unusual and individual situations that may arise–such as those bulleted above, or in the following example. The bulleted situations above obviously would call for brief elementary instructions such as, "You will need to remove your clothing, except for underwear should that feel more comfortable, lie on the bottom sheet, and cover yourself with the sheet/blanket. I will give you a few minutes to make those preparations."

In some instances when I was explaining the clothing procedure to a female client I would be interrupted with, "*EVERYTHING*???" [Note: This type of response indicates a very modest or perhaps fearful individual who may need more assurance because of vulnerability issues (see Emotional Release, Section II)]. For people in this category who are having their first massage, it may be advisable to tell them *each time* you are going to move the sheet/blanket in order to work on a specific area (leg, buttocks, etc.). And especially when you ask them to turn themselves over, state that you will see to it they remain covered as they do so. Remember, anything and everything you can do or say that will allow your clients to be more relaxed will ensure an easier job for you and a more relaxing and beneficial outcome for them.

There have been those times during my pre-massage chat while explaining the procedure, asking if there were any specific areas they preferred longer work on during the massage, etc., when some women would just start undressing! At this point, it is the better part of discretion to say, "Let me leave you to get ready." Even if they replied, "Oh, I don't care … we're both women," I preferred to simply say, "I'll just give you a few minutes," made my exit, and finished our chat after they were under the sheets. However, everyone has their own perspective on this, and it really comes down to what both you and your clients are comfortable with.

In addition: pay attention to what clients may be "telling" you with their body language. Learn to sense what their facial expressions are "saying," and even what they may be trying to tell you by silent osmosis. Be gentle when situations require it, and authoritative when necessary.

COMPETITION AND EGOS
Keep Your Balance

Every human alive needs and enjoys praise; it motivates us to succeed and to work even more diligently at perfecting our skills. It is natural to feel good about yourself and what you are contributing. Yet humans also have the tendency for strong egos, and we run into competitive behaviors in all areas of life. If you know within yourself that you are good at what you do, use that awareness positively. The stronger your self-esteem and confidence in your own Being, the less likely you will become unbalanced by a need to proclaim your worth to others. When you observe that others seem to be boastful in sharing every comment of praise they have received about themselves, simply understand there may be a need or a lack within these people they are not recognizing in themselves.

Once I received a compliment indirectly from a doctor whom I had massaged. At the time I actually was in his office receiving treatment, and he was addressing the massage therapist he'd just instructed to work out trigger points in my body. The doctor mentioned I was also a massage therapist, with "golden hands," to which the other therapist replied, "*Well*, I have *yet* to meet *my* match." A case in point.

Leave your ego out of your work. Be the best of your own potential; that will suffice. Every therapist is going to bring something different and unique to the table.

If some clients do not care for your technique, please understand they are not saying they don't like YOU. If you cannot help them with what it is they are looking for, or you cannot go as deep as their body needs without risk to your own body, refer them to someone who can. This does not mean you are not good or you are lacking in any way as a therapist. It simply means they may be able to benefit from another's technique or skills. We are in business to help people; referring them to someone with skills they need that may be different from yours *IS* helping them!

CONFIDENTIALITY
It Matters

To reiterate an admirable quality of utmost importance, *whatever* is discussed during your time with your clients, whether verbal or written, should be considered absolutely and unequivocally confidential. There may even be clients who do not wish to have *anyone* know they are receiving massage. This is not to be questioned nor judged.

At the grocery store one day I saw one of my clients with two people I assumed to be his wife and little girl. He recognized me and quickly averted his eyes, indicating he preferred not to acknowledge me, so I took his lead and followed along. There was no personal reason between us for his avoidance; i.e., his appointment was for legitimate therapeutic massage, but this reaction was his choice and I respected it. He returned to me for other massages and never mentioned our recognition in the store.

It is always the better part of discretion to allow your clients to make the first acknowledgment when you meet away from your place of business.

I would also extend this courtesy when leaving phone messages as well. Respect that your clients may live with others and would like their private lives to remain confidential.

PERSONAL BAGGAGE
If You're Not Traveling, Leave It At Home

The unspoken rule for every job: don't bring your personal issues to your place of business. Make time before entering your workplace to let go of problems or "mind clutter" that might obstruct your focused attention on your clients. No matter how terrific a massage therapist you may be, we all have our "off" days, and if you are not up to working on people for one reason or another, please do not. This is especially important for massage therapists. By the very hands-on nature of your chosen field, you are not only in people's personal space, you are touching them when they are virtually naked and more vulnerable, and your energies and theirs are being exchanged. They *will* sense if you seem to be out of sync.

I have received massages from people I wished had not gone to work that day. I would rather they had cancelled my appointment than work on me in the condition they were manifesting. It would have been disappointing, but I would have respected their decision. Instead, I could sense their mind and energy were somewhere else and their hands were just going through the motions. And herein lays an important thought for you to keep in mind: your tension is transferable. If you are not balanced in mind/body/spirit, your massages can leave your clients feeling worse than if they had not had the massage–something no one needs!

Your job involves giving–you are in the business of nurturing and taking care of others. In order to do that you must first take care of yourself. Learn to put your issues "on the shelf"; they'll be waiting for you when you return, and the distraction from them will probably serve you well. Assist your clients in this regard by suggesting that they will receive a greater benefit from their massage if they leave whatever might be bothering them outside the door. That if they need, they can "pick it up" on their way out, but for the massage hour you recommend releasing it.

PREJUDICES
Who Needs 'em!

My belief? If you have them, you're in the wrong career. End of story.

PROFESSIONAL
ATHLETES/CELEBRITIES
Get A Grip!

My advice? Leave any feelings you may have of being "star struck" out of the room. People of fame get massages just like the rest of us. You can imagine how much they would prefer a certain semblance of anonymity without being stared at and listening to how much you might admire them. Give your best and respect them as regular human beings.

SHARING YOUR BELIEFS
Others Just May Not Be Interested!

In sharing an unpleasant massage experience one of my clients had, she confided that another therapist had talked constantly during the massage about her own beliefs. She related "how annoying it was to listen that my aura wasn't clear and that my chakras were not aligned."

Always be cautious what you choose to share regarding your beliefs. Keep things very general. The only time I ventured into something more in-depth was when clients talked openly about their own experiences and either asked me about myself or I was comfortable in sharing certain personal information.

Take your clients' hints. Pay attention to their clues. Use your intuition. Professional boundaries take precedence in a professional setting.

TAKING THINGS PERSONALLY
Who, ME???

Unfortunately there are people "out there" who are miserable and can't wait to bring you into that world with them. Usually (at least we hope!) this is unconscious behavior, but whether it is or not does not make it easier to handle. We all have encountered individuals who are rude, irritated, "got up on the wrong side of the bed," or what-have-you. The good thing is that you don't have to associate with them if you choose not to–*unless* of course, they're scheduled to be on *your* table!

How to smooth ruffled feathers? Begin with yourself … deep breathing is recommended as a good starting point. Remove yourself emotionally from the behavior and/or comments. Or, put another way, become an observer of your own situation. If after suggesting your client relax in the moment, clear distractive mental thoughts, breathe deeply, and/or focus on music in the background, you see that any benefits to your client from massage are simply not going to be possible, you may wish to address your client, explaining that his/her agitation is interfering with any possibility of experiencing any benefits from the massage. Should the situation become inappropriate or abusive, simply end the massage. If you work at a facility and feel it would be best for a manager to handle the situation, by all means, excuse yourself and involve the manager! But if the situation subsides, brush it mentally aside, knowing you handled yourself as well as could be expected under the circumstances.

Remember, the behavior of others rarely has anything to do with you; it has everything to do with them. Not taking things personally will be a learning opportunity you will face many times during your career. Use it to your benefit.

TIPS
The $ Kind

Tipping has become a part of life in all areas of the working world for every possible service, yet some people choose to give and some people do not. In the massage world, it also depends on the type of environment: medical clients generally do not tip, whereas salon and spa clients are more apt to express their appreciation in that fashion.

This kind of "tip" might serve you well to consider: if your thoughts are focused more on what amount of tip you may receive rather than how you might be able to help your client, you will project a different energy than what you might wish your client to feel. It is best to have no expectations in this regard. Then if you do receive a tip, you will have a nice surprise! And if you do not, you still will have the personal fulfillment of a massage well given.

WHEN TO SAY NO
Absolutely, Unequivocally

Upon arriving at the home of a first-time client I was met at the door by her daughter, who explained her mother was not feeling well. I asked questions about what the problem might be when I noticed the woman sitting on the steps. Introducing myself, I sat with her. Gradually she shared that surgery had been performed on her legs two weeks previously and she was now experiencing "tension" in them. I asked her many more questions before urging her to call her doctor immediately. She said she would, after the massage, and begged me to skip her legs and work on her back, stating it was "killing" her and she "couldn't take the pain." She even told me her doctor had said, "Massage is fine."

For a situation such as this you have but *one option*: say no and stick to it! Her problem may have been nothing unusual under the circumstances of that particular surgery, but you *must consider the risk* to your client–and yourself–should the opposite be the case.

When in doubt or dealing with any unknown, it's *always* NO!

SECTION II

COME OUT, COME OUT, WHEREVER YOU ARE
This Is No Time For Hide-And-Seek

There has been that rare occasion when a client takes an extremely long time to come out of the massage room.

When I was managing a massage business, a therapist came to me stating that the gentleman she had just worked on had not come out of the room she had left 10 minutes ago. She had knocked twice without receiving a reply. I went to the door and knocked, announcing at the same time that I was the manager and was wondering if everything was okay. No response. I then stated it had been 15 minutes and we needed the room for the next client. It sounded like the client was getting dressed, and I waited for an answer but none came. I then knocked harder and restated in a louder voice, "Sir, is everything all right? We're becoming a bit concerned about you." He then stated he would be right out. I waited with the therapist until he opened the door, escorted him to the front, and waited while he checked out and left the establishment.

We all discussed our assumptions about this person's behavior, but since there were no clues from him or in the massage room that would indicate what the problem might have been, we came to the conclusion that some situations are simply unresolvable.

DISSATISFIED CLIENTS
You Can't Please Everyone All The Time

Working as a manager at a massage clinic, one day I received an "I want to speak to the manager" call from a woman who had left only 30 minutes previously. I listened as this obviously very upset woman explained that she had never had such a terrible massage. "I am a regular client," she spoke. "I have been loyal to your establishment and I have never been so disappointed in my life." An apology was extended, I assured her that her call was appreciated, and personally offered to give her a free massage. I did not feel it was necessary in this instance to share the woman's call with the therapist in question. She had worked at this clinic for several years, had many clients who loved her work, and there was nothing to be gained.

It may be difficult if anything like this ever happens and you *are* aware that your client did not particularly care for your massage. But perhaps it will be helpful to understand that not everyone is going to like a particular touch, technique, style, or energy. It may be a blow to your ego, but remember there are clients who adore your work. You *can* take each unpleasant comment personally and be miserable, yet that is not very self-serving.

As massage therapists, we thrive on three little words: "That was *great!*" There were times when I left a massage wondering whether certain of my clients liked my work. Some never made a comment one way or another. There are simply too many variables involved in dealing with personalities to be able to please everyone during your career. Maturing into the place where you feel good about yourself and your abilities without having to count on your clients stroking you is a very balanced state of mind to strive for.

MASSAGE CLIENT EXPERTS
Who's Who Here?

Believe it or not, there are some individuals who believe they know how to do your job better than you, and may even give you instructions about your massaging techniques from your table! As annoying and/or insulting as this may seem, remember to keep your emotional balance. Politely respond with a non-committal comment such as, "Thanks; I've got it covered," or "Maybe I'll try that sometime," even though you may *want* to say something else! Stay composed and just carry on.

Be cautious not to confuse this type of comment with one given by a client who asks you to repeat a move you've done before, or express how good a certain technique feels.

I had a regular client that asked me if I'd try something she'd liked about another massage she had experienced. My first reaction was surprise, but I quickly came to realize that it was something she enjoyed and, if I could make her feel better during our time together, then it was something I could certainly try. Because I was willing and open to trying something new, I learned a new technique from my client. She continued to see me regularly and it became a joke between us–how *she* taught me!

PROTECTIVE BOUNDARIES
Personal Roadblocks

Have you ever noticed a sense of "invasion" if someone gets too close to you? Sometimes you may feel comfortable yet other times somewhat uncomfortable, but why? If you observe people, you might see them either back away from or move closer to others, depending on what they are feeling. As we become more learned about the anatomy of our physical body, we also learn about the layers of energy that surround the body as well. We come to realize that anything and everything has a vibrational energy. Our energy fields provide us with a sense of awareness similar to intuition. When someone steps into *your* energy field, you sense *their* energies in your "space" immediately, as both vibrational fields automatically begin interacting. The reaction can be either positive or negative.

It is a wise idea to find ways to avoid being susceptible to any negativity you may encounter. As massage therapists we are literally and constantly "hands-on" with a variety of energies. Protecting one's own energy field is important to your well-being.

How does one go about protecting oneself? Setting boundaries. Making decisions as to what topics of conversation you may or may not choose to talk about with a client. Knowing when to say No. Defining your standard of values and abiding by them. Learning how to observe without emotion. How to speak with clarity and firmness when necessary. Keeping physically fit. Living and eating healthy. Thinking positively.

SERVICE OUTSIDE YOUR EXPERTISE
Expanding Your Abilities

Many times when clients call to schedule appointments they know to specify the type of massage they wish to receive. Many times … not always! One of my clients had not mentioned during our pre-massage chat that she was interested in having energy work instead of a regular massage. If she had, it would not have been necessary for me to leave the room since one can remain fully clothed for energy work. When I re-entered she had removed her clothing and was lying on the table; it was then she requested an "energy massage."

While my training had included a short class on energy work, at that time in my career I did not feel particularly confident enough charging someone for an hour's worth! Explaining that I was not comfortable with giving her a full hour of energy work because I had only worked using that technique for a short time, she asked if I would do what I knew. Though I was reluctant, I agreed, and was amazed that the hour seemed to zoom by. As you might imagine I, myself, was not feeling thoroughly satisfied, but my client praised me and thanked both the receptionist and me for "a wonderful hour."

"The moral of this story," as the saying goes, is no matter what the outcome may be, if clients ask you for a particular technique even though you have been honest and explained your situation and feelings, give it a try–it's how you learn (unless of course you have had no training and/or are completely uncomfortable). They may be satisfied, they may not, but at least you had been up-front and offered them the choice.

TARDINESS
They're Late, They're Late, For A Very Important Date

Get ready! You will have them all:

- Clients who show up at the wrong time but "*really* need a massage" …
- Clients who are late and you can't give them a full hour because you have other clients stacked behind them …
- Clients who are **so** late you can't give them even a fraction of the time …
- Clients who got stuck in traffic …
- Clients whose children were late getting out of school …
- … and many, many others….

You will have situations where people are rushing in 10, 20, even 30 minutes late yet are still expecting their full hour, or will call 20 minutes before their scheduled appointment and cancel at the proverbial last minute. Being aware of your options in handling these types of situations is the key to minimizing your stress. I've done all sorts of finagling in order to please clients. I've switched and swapped and squeezed appointments in an attempt to accommodate everyone. When you're working on a tight schedule, this can be quite frustrating. Being understanding and graciously accepting apologies is one thing; continually allowing others not to respect your time and energy is another.

I've also had my share of staying late to accommodate clients. In one circumstance a woman became quite upset because she claimed my boss had obviously written down the wrong time on the scheduling sheet. I did not argue with her about who was right or wrong in scheduling–there's no sense in getting involved in irrelevant bickering about an unknown. Instead I offered her the option of either receiving a half-hour massage right then or returning in 1.5 hours for a full hour massage. Unrelenting, she reiterated that it was my boss's fault for putting down the wrong time. I then offered her a 10% discount for this misunderstanding. She finally began to settle down, came back later, and we had a wonderful hour. I had made a personal decision in this situation to take less money simply to keep her coming back. I received no "Thank You" for staying late or reducing my fee. Unfortunately and for some reason, massage clients seem not to realize that this is our livelihood, nor do they consider the therapist's time nor salary in a prorated hour. This type of situation is just something you have to work through with each individual. And even then, sometimes there is just nothing you can do to appease a client who is determined to be upset.

Some spas or other massage establishments make it a standard practice to take credit card numbers when scheduling appointments, informing each person they will be charged 50% or 100% of the fee for a no-show, and enforcing that rule according to their discretion. Some massage establishments allow a grace period and then will schedule your time with another client. This is a considerate gesture for the therapist in that you will still be paid for that time *and* you are not faced with having to confront your late client. Some businesses have a "No-Fault Policy" and may choose to be very strict about it or never uphold it. If you're working for someone else, make yourself aware of these types of policies/procedures so you know where you stand and whether or not you would receive support for any particular decision you may be called upon to make.

You can request not to see a particular client again if you are working for a spa or other business environment. However, if you are dealing with a personal client it may be a more difficult situation because naturally you don't want to lose a client. I would suggest doing all you possibly can to make it work. Give people the benefit of the doubt until such time as they abuse even that.

No matter what your working environment, if clients develop the habit of arriving late, you should find a way to politely discuss with them the inconveniences it causes both of you. You may wish to include the fact that you allow a specified amount of time for each client for the most beneficial relaxation and necessary muscle work, and if someone is consistently tardy it makes it difficult or impossible to achieve that. Suggest their leaving for the appointment destination earlier, allowing more time to account for traffic or weather delays, or scheduling an appointment at a more convenient time or another day of the week.

On the other hand, certainly there are those times when tardiness simply can't be helped. *The consistency of certain clients to be late versus justifiable reasons for being late are what you have to consider in each individual situation.*

UNPLEASANT AND/OR UNDESIRABLE CLIENTS
It Takes All Kinds

I had become acquainted with another massage therapist at a continuing education class we had both attended. Although we seemed to be compatible and a friendship began between us, as she shared more of her life with me during the next few weeks I began to feel uncomfortable with certain aspects of her personality and characteristics. While I certainly did not want to hurt her feelings, I decided it would be best to back away from furthering the relationship. I did so, but she pursued my attention, often leaving messages on my various phone services more than once daily. She scheduled a massage with me at my place of work, which I did not know about until I saw her name on my daily list.

Now, if you do not wish to give any particular massage, it is your right and your option to decline. Understand that should you ever do this, the reason you present to your employer must show appropriate cause. Should at any time you believe it would be harmful to you in some respect, then that is what you state. If you are self-employed, of course you would never schedule someone you wish to avoid, yet you still would need to have a feasible and inoffensive (as possible) reason to offer without possibly creating a greater problem.

Another client, a male, came religiously to the spa where I worked every Thursday evening at the same hour. He presented himself as being nice, successful, and confident. After about 10 minutes on the table, I realized his ego was going to be a domineering factor during his massage. His conversations were nonstop throughout all future massages and the focus always centered around how much money he made, which of his very expensive cars he was planning to use that evening, etc. He was not intolerable, but he was rather boastful–*and* he was literally talking himself out of a more relaxing and beneficial hour of massage. I reasoned that perhaps it helped him to express himself in this way. It was not my job to determine otherwise. He continued to come weekly for months and I continued to allow him his "ego therapy" by listening until I left that particular establishment.

It was a great lesson in tolerance and patience!

SECTION III

BAD BREATH
The Non-Clinical Name For Halitosis

Inhaling another's exhales can be rather unpleasant at times, especially when you are working close to your client's face. My worst scenario in this category was when I was massaging a gentleman that must have had garlic for lunch and then smoked a cigar afterwards. He would consistently take very deep breaths and (for some reason) kept turning his head toward me to exhale, completely unaware that his relaxation technique was causing me discomfort. My chosen line of defense was to continue working normally while attempting to move out of "breath's way" without causing a distraction when he began his exhalation.

You can try positioning your body opposite from the direction your clients are breathing by turning their head to one side as if this was a normal part of your massage technique. I later learned the very simple technique of keeping mints handy in my office. When you greet your clients, take a mint yourself and offer one to them. This works fabulously! No one is offended and all grounds have been covered.

Always keep in mind that *you* are breathing near your *clients'* faces, too. (It will keep you humble!)

BODY HAIR
It Can Be Anywhere And Everywhere

There can be many different variations in people concerning this topic. Generally speaking, our society has deemed body hair more or less undesirable and a majority of people do prefer the appearance of smooth skin. Yet there are many of both genders who either prefer their natural state or simply are of the genetic heritage to have an abundance–and some may be embarrassed by this and some may not. Nevertheless, you will undoubtedly encounter some of them on your massage table.

One of my experiences in this regard was with a man whose back was covered with hair so thick I could not see his skin beneath it. As a fairly new massage therapist, I wondered, "How am I going to do this???" I soon realized that lotion was not the answer, but found oil to be my best friend in the moment! If and when you encounter such a situation, start with a small amount of oil and smooth out any knots that may occur with more oil. It was somewhat difficult and I felt as though the poor man had been "slathered"–or perhaps anointed! But, "All's Well That Ends Well," and it had!

Note: Friction isn't really recommended or possible under these circumstances!

BODY ODOR
Thexe Axe Ways To Avoid The Pungency!

One of the most common situations you may encounter, this subject has a variety of possibilities. Adopting non-judgment in this and other sensitive areas will serve you well. People are often immune to their own body odor, and there are those few who struggle to control this aspect of their physicality. Or those who may have such severe allergies to anything scented or that contains certain ingredients may simply avoid deodorants and soaps, so be sure to give your clients the benefit of the doubt.

You will undoubtedly experience an occasional yet reasonably mild whiff of body odor that is actually quite normal, and then there will be times it will seem as if the odor is coming from every pore of the body, capable of permeating the entire room. This may occur more noticeably in people who regularly eat spicy foods or those who are particularly heavy smokers of cigarettes and/or cigars. The human body will expunge the odor of illnesses, medications or other toxins through the skin. And then there are those people who simply have different values concerning bathing hygiene.

I had a woman client who was undergoing chemotherapy treatment for cancer. She desperately needed the nurturing touch of massage and, although there were moments that the odors being released were intensified *because* of the massage and were difficult for me to handle, I made a personal choice to keep working with her weekly. There are some things that are just more important and soul-satisfying than the comfort of a pleasing scent. But such a situation is always a matter of choice–one that you should make based upon what your circumstances and tolerance levels are.

Those are a few of the problems in this aspect of massage; following are a few suggestions that you may wish to consider, remembering all the while that *you* are the one in control!

- If situations of this nature are tolerable, then carry on. If, on the other hand, it becomes too unpleasant, you might gently move your client's arms closer to the body as if it were a natural position for the way you choose to massage. You might also avoid lifting the arms at all.

- If this massage is a one-time client, then you just need to place that experience in your "That wasn't the easiest, but I survived" category.

- If this is a problem with regular clients and the odor is more than tolerable, you might want to state the benefits of bathing before a session by suggesting, "Water relaxes us and prepares the body for a more beneficial massage experience. Perhaps we could schedule any future massages at a time that would allow you to include a relaxing bath or shower beforehand." (Be Creative!)

- You may wish to adopt a standard procedure of asking ALL clients to wash their feet with a warm towel before the massage, or you could warm a towel and wipe the feet during the massage, treating it as part of your routine. Make sure the towel is warm–and never scrub; massage the foot *with* the towel. Prepare your clients before applying the towel so they will not be caught off guard.

- Have a subtly scented candle lit in your massage room/area.

- Turn on a fan to circulate the air.

- There are gloves available specifically for massage therapists, though I have never used them. You may wish to try them and want to have some available, "just in case."

- Use a naturally scented spray in your room between clients.

- After the massage, swab the massage table (as usual) with a cleansing agent/rubbing alcohol, change the sheets, and scrub your hands.

Above all, no matter what the circumstances, always treat your clients with kindness and sensitivity.

CHATTERBOXES
Talk Isn't Cheap!

It is guaranteed you will have people on your table who just cannot stop talking. The very ambiance of your massage area sets the perfect stage: soft music playing in the background, dimmed lighting, a peaceful atmosphere, privacy, they are being catered to, and they have your undivided attention! They are there to relax and to *be* relaxed, yet those who "live in the fast lane" may have difficulty changing gears without a gradual unwinding. And because they really can't move about on your table to release energy, their only recourse is to talk.

After several minutes, if any of your clients seem to be rambling incessantly and insignificantly, suggest they take a deep breath in that moment and begin to relax. Ask them questions about how the massage is feeling in an attempt to get them to focus on what is happening with their physical body in the present moment. Sometimes this will work and sometimes it will not. Regardless, let your hands speak relaxation and calm, whether the client can stop chattering or not.

Another reason people may choose not to stop talking could be their need to express. They may feel safe with your energy and recognize you as someone to whom they can vent. I worked with a woman that had terminal cancer who consistently talked on and off during our many sessions together. I never attempted to stop or interrupt her because I realized she actually was releasing feelings she could not express honestly to friends and family. She needed me to listen. I listened, and left feeling privileged to be so trusted.

On the other hand, I have also had clients tell me how annoying it has been for them to receive massage when their *therapist* was talking. One client shared that another massage therapist she had seen talked the whole hour about her boyfriend and what he had done to annoy her the past evening. This is a definite "Red Flag" message for all massage therapists to take to heart!

My suggested rule of thumb? If a client asks a question, answer it appropriately. If it is about something personal and is outside the comfort level of your boundaries, respond with those words. Always use discretion in the amount of information you reveal about yourself. I very seldom ask my clients questions about anything other than massage-related topics, especially when they are on the table. Again, use discretion.

CLIENTS OF SIZE
A Delicate Balance

One's weight or height usually is not considered much of an issue in massage. However, an extra hundred or more pounds or several inches can present difficulties when a person of size is not able to fit comfortably on your table.

Although first impressions of having to work on an extremely large person may seem daunting, we each have the opportunity to be grateful for the experience it will provide for us. It serves us well to recognize the painful stereotypes people of excess weight are faced with and what they must have to overcome just to receive a massage. Some larger size clients may tend to feel uncomfortable in a naked state, or just having someone touching them, and others will tend to be quite the opposite. How your opinions come across to them will tell them whether or not you are a safe person and can be trusted with their vulnerability.

In a society where appearances seem to mean everything, I had a tremendous amount of respect for a woman of approximately 400 pounds whose arms and legs hung off my table. Situations of this type do not allow the therapist much room to work against the support of the table and can be physically draining. Her skin was thick and I wondered how she could possibly be feeling the benefits of my work, but I soon realized that such a thought is limiting because *massage therapists do more for their clients than massage them*. It became obvious to me during her massage that she needed to have a very nurturing touch, one that spoke of acceptance and non-judgment.

This particular client on my table requested a very light pressure, which relieved my concern in that regard because I had realized it would not be possible for me to provide her with a deep-tissue massage. Should this not be possible for you to do and a person of size requests a deep-tissue massage, however, you might simply state that your physical structure and strength prohibits you from providing that service for him/her, that you could offer a relaxing massage, or would honor their prerogative to seek a massage therapist who is more capable in this regard.

One experience I had was with a first-time client that stood 6'9''. He had not mentioned his height to the receptionist so we had no time to prepare … even though I'm not sure at that time what we would have done. We had no table extensions or footrests available so I basically did the best I could. We talked about it beforehand and he knew what he was in for. He had "experienced this before" and knew his feet would hang off. I made the massage as comfortable as I could using the headrest and pillows to "extend" the table.

If you tend to have tall or large clients, it may be in your best interest to invest in the table extensions, side arms, or extra wide tables that can be purchased to make your work easier and more comfortably accommodate your clients.

Treating them with the greatest of respect will leave their self-esteem unharmed.

"DON'T MESS UP MY HAIR/MAKEUP!"
A Direct Quote!

This "request" was always perplexing to me because of its restrictive nature and the fact that a portion of benefit from the massage was lost before I even began! It was also somewhat amusing since I wasn't sure how I was expected to use oil and massage deep into the neck, yet avoid getting even a strand of hair out of place!

One of my female clients requested that I use oil but did not want any to get in her hair. I explained I would do the best I could, but if I could use lotion it would be easier to avoid any disruption. She wasn't crazy about the idea at first but eventually consented. Should you encounter this situation, try wrapping a towel loosely around the head while massaging the back, and avoid working on the neck while the person is supine. If this becomes a regular request, you may want to have a few lightweight shower caps available–just in case. Use a towel to rub off any excess residue left on the skin after you are finished with the massage. For those clients who prefer oil, switch from lotion to oil after you've finished with the area around the head.

Suggest to those clients who are concerned about their makeup that they turn their head to one side to lessen any smearing of the cosmetics. (Obviously the face would not be included in the massage.) Be aware that some cosmetics are difficult to get out of sheets and towels. When pressing the face into the face cradle, they will inevitably have most of the makeup residue on the cover … it's just a fact of massage life! Please don't be shy in informing clients should they have mascara smeared down their face; some people don't always check before leaving the office.

Just do the best you can, however seemingly impossible the request.

EMOTIONAL RELEASE
A Healthy Thing, Indeed

Many people simply do not have the awareness that muscles hold memory. Not the kind our brains hold, but *physical* memory of experiences from our past that were traumatizing to one degree or another and "stored" in some area of the body. Massaging those areas–even years later–can trigger the same feelings and emotions from the original injury or trauma, whether it was mental, emotional, physical, or spiritual.

Often clients will suddenly and spontaneously find themselves weeping–slightly to uncontrollably–or laughing as these emotions are released. These clients are likely to be quite surprised and probably embarrassed, and some will apologize. Assure them there is no need to apologize, that this happens often and is just another healing benefit of massage. Explain what it is that is happening and why, and encourage them not to try to control their reaction but to follow it through, to "let it all out," even though they may not be able to fathom what the association is at that moment. As it rises from a subconscious state to a conscious state, the connection to the original trauma may "click," though that is not necessary for the release to be therapeutic.

Stay aware of how emotional your client's response is and react accordingly; i.e., continuing the massage, stopping, or leaving the room. If it seems appropriate, ask if your client would like a moment alone. If the answer is no, keep your hands gently on their shoulders as a silent gesture of support. It often helps just to know they are not alone in this type of experience. You should be able to resume massaging within a few minutes. Use your intuition in this type of situation.

Besides always having a box of tissues at hand, your job is to remain grounded and calmly and gently do your best to facilitate what could be a very healing experience for your client.

EYES WIDE OPEN
The Better To See You With, My Dear

For whatever the reason, from the moment I started with his massage, a first-time male client was fixated with staring at me and following my every move with his eyes. This became rather disconcerting, so in my calmest voice I told him, "Relax, and close your eyes." He would, for about three seconds–then his eyelids would spring open and his eyes continued to follow my movements. I kept repeating, "Relax, just close your eyes," but the staring was relentless. Realizing I was fighting a losing battle, and beginning to feel rather uneasy, I turned him over–which, of course, put him face down, ending the "stalking" sensation—and spent the remainder of the hour working on his back.

Whether he was concerned with what I might do to him in his perceived vulnerable state or this behavior was natural to him–or *whatever* was going on–remains a mystery. Regardless, I felt it necessary to make it known that his obsessive staring was uncomfortable and I was taking control of the situation.

The point here is to listen to your gut feelings. Anything that causes you to be intimidated, uncomfortable, or simply question the motive of someone's actions is reason enough to change the circumstances and regain a balance in as normal and polite a way as possible.

FLATULENCE
To Be Or Not To Be (Embarrassed), That Is The Question

The generating of gaseous elements in the alimentary canal–such a normal function of the human physical body–has gotten a bad rap! In many cultures bodily functions that create a sound when expelled are acceptable without so much as a thought. But this particular and very normal physical occurrence often causes reactions of instant humiliation and embarrassment to the perpetrator and awkwardness to all those around. Now when you think about it in these terms, isn't that *interesting!*?!?

Scientific explanations notwithstanding, however, when the body is relaxed and there is pressure on our gluteus muscles–as during a massage–this bodily function tends to occur more often! So now it becomes a situation "up close and personal," as the saying goes, especially if neither you nor your client happen to be talking in that moment (the greater the silence, the greater the embarrassment), or should an odor accompany the sound and you should happen to be "in the vicinity"–which is even more humiliating to your client, not to mention a bit unpleasant for you.

That's the physical. Now take a moment to realize what it is any one of your clients may be experiencing emotionally and mentally in this situation. Whenever we are feeling "less-than", which is a form of fear (and you *know* they'd rather not be sharing this moment), stress occurs in the body. This causes the muscles to tighten up and the heart rate to increase, which means it's now up to you to calm them down and relax them in the interest of giving them a satisfying massage! Whew! What a cycle, huh?

No, I have not been exempt from situations in this category! From my experience, there are two ways your clients will handle the moment: they will say something, or they will say nothing. The first time I encountered this circumstance *I* chose to say nothing because I didn't *know* what to say, but I did know I did not want to make the matter worse for my client. One woman's reaction was to say, "OH! Excuse me!" A simple comment such as, "It happens–we're all human" or, "It just means you're relaxed" should serve to dissolve your client's embarrassment immediately.

There was another occasion when I was concentrating intensely on deep-tissue work to the lower back when my client's gas escaped; it startled me and I jumped ... she was embarrassed, and so was I for my reaction. She apologized and I answered with, "Oh, no worries–it happens all the time," and nothing more was said. Usually the "release" happens while they are lying prone–which makes it easier for you, considering even a slight smile on your part may be offensive, and offending someone is not so good for business! Aside from being an aid in relaxation, having calming music playing in the background will diminish any impact of embarrassment simply because there is something else to focus on–another audible distraction–in the moment.

One gentleman client completely ignored that it had happened. He had fallen asleep during the massage and been wakened by this "situation," whereupon he quickly proceeded to clear his throat in an attempt to mask that the sound had actually come from a different part of his body than where he was wishing it had!

One thing I can guarantee ... if you are a massage therapist, you *will* encounter this awkward moment, and not just once! *How you react will make the difference between night and day to your client in their vulnerability of the moment.* So work with yourself; if you are inclined to giggle in these instances, find a way to handle your reactions before the situation occurs. Let's face it: awkwardness and embarrassment are the emotions that *cause* people to laugh, snicker, or giggle in order to release those very emotions when they don't know what else to do. Changing your mental perception concerning this very normal bodily function is really your best defense against a reaction that can only cause you and your client additional or unnecessary embarrassment. You'll be a pro at it in no time! And a polite one, at that!

Summary: If an embarrassing situation happens, always treat your clients during and following the massage with the attitude that implies this type of thing happens to the best of us. Make sure they can sense your sincerity about their comfort level and welfare when their session is finished; look them straight in the eye. Take the time to talk with them about non-related subjects. If they should still be feeling any awkwardness, at least you will have done your part in mending any permanent embarrassment.

HAIR PLUGS, TOUPEES, AND WIGS
Props To Be Handled With Care

Though it is usually noticeable when a person has added a hairpiece to their physical body, always scan your client for this possibility. Some may nonchalantly remove a toupee or wig and place it with their clothing. Most people in this category will mention the fact to you and let you know whether or not you are to include the scalp in their massage, yet there is always the occasional instance where it is never mentioned, perhaps because some massage therapists never include the head/scalp in their routine. My choice in such cases was simply to avoid the scalp, eliminating any possible embarrassment to my client.

I worked for one chiropractor who happened to have hair plugs of the more obvious type. When he asked me to give him a massage, my immediate assumption was to avoid his head/scalp, but he actually requested that area.

In all such situations, work very gently and do not pull!

HAIR SPRAY
And Sometimes Lots Of It!

Depending on the type of environment you will be working in, some individuals will want the scalp massage and some will not. Those who wish to include it usually make their requests during the pre-massage chat when you both discuss where the focus will be, the condition of their body, and any special problems they may be experiencing.

As I began one particular massage by working on the face and neck of a woman who had requested I include her scalp, I studied her *heavily* sprayed hair in an attempt to figure out where I might be able to penetrate it with my fingers in order to *reach* her scalp. Realizing it just *wasn't* going to happen, I placed my hands on *top* of her hair and did the best I could. By the time I was done, my hands felt like they did back in kindergarten when I'd poured Elmer's glue on my fingers and let it set about five minutes! It was not the only occasion in which I encountered this minor difficulty!

If it looks as though hairspray or gel might be in excess, you may want to suggest, "I would be able to do a better job if you would brush through your hair; that way we could avoid any pulling that may occur." Again, even including the scalp under these circumstances is your choice.

I recommend having moist towelettes among your supplies for such situations!

OIL SPILLS
On Humans

If you are a therapist who chooses to use oil for your massages, you might have an occasion when a drop or two–or a downright spill–may accidentally "escape" from your hands or the bottle onto an area of a client's body. The worst scenario would be if the oil was to land on your client's face. Should such an embarrassing situation occur, and especially if it occurs at the outset of the massage, unfortunately it could tend to set the wrong tone. *Good preventive techniques are to be cautious when using your pump, **never** pour anything while your hands are over your client, and lubricate your hands away from your client's body.*

However, *if* it happens, and *wherever* it falls, apologize and gently remove the excess oil. The situation will be easier to disguise if it happens on someone's back. But even so, remember we are all more aware of sensations during massage, so it is most likely even a drop would be felt and be a bit startling.

Also keep in mind that mistakes happen. No one is exempt.

PHYSICAL DEFORMITIES
Awareness Equals Preparation

This experience is shared with the greatest respect for my client and all others whose daily lives are challenged with physical differences. Your responsibility is not only to provide them with a great massage, but also silent acceptance and appreciation for what their personal journeys must entail. The clients about whom I write presented me with the gift of education concerning the realities of others.

While working at a salon, I greeted a somewhat shorter than most woman with long hair who was wearing a turtle-neck sweater and escorted her to my massage room. We discussed all the prerequisites regarding illness, surgeries, medication, etc. She informed me she had received massages before and was not there with any specific problems; she was there to "relax." I explained all the minor details and left the room. When I returned she was tucked under the sheets face down. I walked over and began my routine.

Moving the sheet down, I gently lifted her hair away from her back. To my absolute shock I noticed this woman had a deformity I had never known as possible: her hairline went across the top of her shoulders. She actually did not have a neck; her head was literally sitting on her shoulders. This was a difficult moment of realization for me and had totally caught me off guard. Yet wanting to spare her embarrassment or hurt feelings, I quickly composed myself and proceeded with the massage.

On another occasion a gentleman walked into my clinic and I could see at first glance that his right arm was shorter and smaller in size than his left. I greeted him and we sat down to talk. He told me about the accident that had occurred and what I should expect in regard to range of motion, etc. He was very matter-of-fact and had no difficulty discussing the situation. We kept the communication open during the actual treatment and it was a nice exchange, leaving one of us feeling relaxed, and the other satisfied about being able to help–without having been caught off guard!

I am not sure why the woman chose not to mention her condition; perhaps because it was so normal for her. The key message here is simply to be aware that there are those who may appear slightly different in some way or another, but who nonetheless have the same, or perhaps even more sensitive feelings. Although we can't always completely prepare ourselves for any given situation, just having the knowledge of such possibilities will hopefully soften any experience you may encounter.

RELAXATION AND YOUR
TUMMY'S REACTION
Talk To Me, Baby

When one is receiving massage, the digestive system, as well as the rest of the body, begins to relax, which may cause "tummy gurgles." This is such a normal reaction, yet I have come across only a few individuals that haven't been embarrassed when this occurs.

When you are confronted with this situation, just let your client know it's a normal response to relaxation.

Now to the therapist! There have been times when my own tummy had independently decided to let my client know it wanted sustenance (impatient organ that it can be!), or would, in its satisfaction of having been recently fed, gurgle with the sounds of digestion. "Excuse me," is all that need be said. Sometimes they'll respond, other times they will not.

You may want to keep little snacks to nibble on between clients—nothing with an offensive or lingering odor, but something substantial to keep your tummy from having to announce you have gone beyond its feeding time! I have learned from experience to allow at least 20 minutes (if possible) for my system to digest and settle after a meal before beginning a massage.

SWEATING
Water, Water, Everywhere

The natural body function of perspiring can bring a few special challenges for a massage therapist. Working on a perspiring body simply is not the most enjoyable feeling, but the greater problem is that it is nearly impossible to attain the friction required to massage. Neither you nor your client will enjoy your hour together unless you are prepared for such a situation. The good news is that there *are* ways to deal with this slippery dilemma.

I've welcomed several clients who had just finished working out and even showered, but had not given themselves any time to cool off. Some even have arrived wiping their head with a towel, stating, "It was a great workout!" I asked them to take a few minutes just to breathe deeply and relax, and that I would return with some water for them. Even five minutes will allow a body to cool down sufficiently.

Other times you will encounter people whose bodies simply produce more perspiration than is the norm. It may be because this is simply what their bodies do, or it is possible they may be feeling anxious or uncomfortable about any number of things. You can't always know what's going on in another person's mind/body. Keep extra hand towels available for such occasions. Pat or gently wipe off each area of the body as you move through the massage. If you act as though this is a part of your regular routine, it is unlikely they will even notice what you are doing. Or if they do, they will undoubtedly be silently grateful that you are able to handle what otherwise might be a cause of embarrassment for them. As they relax more during the massage, the situation may even correct itself.

THE EFFECTS OF DEEP SLEEP
Lullaby And Good Night

Occasionally when someone is deeply relaxed and sleeping, one of those noisy little happenings known as snoring can be quite noticeably loud. There have been times when the decibels emanating from my table became so intense that I was not without a small grin, wondering if others could hear my client.

Then there is the other sound that is called a snort that very definitely gets its name because of the sound made when one's nasal/throat passage is blocked in some way. Snorting will often waken the client abruptly and, realizing what has happened, they usually feel embarrassed and will verbally excuse themselves, in which case you can put them at ease with a simple statement about it "not being a problem; it happens often." More often, however, are the attempts to cover the fact of the snort having occurred by coughing, which is best handled by saying nothing.

There may be a time or two when you have clients who become so relaxed that they just cannot seem to wake up! If you know a client is sleeping when the massage is finished, touch a shoulder and gently say the massage is over, to take a few moments before getting up, and meet you outside after dressing. You might wait a moment or two to make sure you were heard and the person begins to stir. After leaving the room, if it seems there are no sounds of movement, after a reasonable amount of time knock softly on the door, asking if everything is okay. I've had those who had gone back to sleep waken again, quite apologetic. A time or two I actually have had to actually go back into the room to waken someone, sometimes having to press a little harder than my gentle nudge to be effective. In those cases many have come out of the room making some remark about my having put them to sleep, thank me for such a relaxing time, or a simple "I needed that...."

It may feel awkward the first few times having to waken a stranger, but as long as you're polite you can only feel complimented for having provided such a relaxing touch that someone felt safe enough to get some undoubtedly needed R&R.

TICKLISH SITUATIONS
A Not-So-Funny Predicament

Being ticklish is a more common "affliction" than you may realize. Those who happen to have a sensitivity to being touched in certain areas of the body require delicate handling. While these people find it difficult not to flinch, jump, or giggle during a massage, there are ways to make their experience a relaxing one.

The feet seem to win the prize for being the most ticklish area of the body, hands down! There *are* tolerance levels to be dealt with. Your ticklish clients may mention their sensitivity to you, but if they do not tell you to avoid their feet, you can usually find a pressure that will be suitable. Some ticklish people find deep pressure to be easier to tolerate, yet others prefer a lighter pressure. Communicate with them; they may be ready to try, and they may not. But if you can help them over this hurdle, they, too, will be able to feel the benefits of a good foot massage.

One of my clients told me she was ticklish the first time I saw her, but I had no idea she was referring to her entire body. I could barely touch her skin–lightly *or* deeply. She seemed very uncomfortable and it was extremely difficult for me to keep any kind of flow with someone who was constantly jerking and giggling. I felt badly for her; I wanted so much for her to relax that I silently committed to the challenge to keep trying. Perhaps the techniques I used will be helpful to you. I asked her to focus on her breathing, and gently touched her skin in a "safe" (less sensitive) place, making sure to touch with my whole hand, firmly but not deeply. I consciously watched her facial expressions and became aware when she felt the tickles coming on, coaching her to take a deep breath every time she felt the urge to laugh. Eventually she was able to do that herself.

Usually I took advantage of her deep breaths to move to another area of her body. We made it through the massage. She ultimately trusted the touch of my hands and even experienced full hours without as much as a giggle. She was a regular client for years.

Don't give up on your clients. They are there voluntarily to relax and unwind, and your job is to find a way to help them do that. It's up to you to be in tune with each individual you work on. In some cases being ticklish is a sign of deep, pent-up sadness or pain [see Emotional Release, Section III]. With that possibility in mind, instead of becoming frustrated or annoyed, view their sensitivity as a challenge to give them the gift of relaxation. That will be your reward.

SECTION IV

ACCIDENTAL EXPOSURE
Oops!

Occasionally a female client's sheet may slip away from her breasts during the massage. If your client is completely relaxed she may not notice
to correct it herself; do not interrupt, and when you can work it naturally
into the massage, gently re-drape the sheet. A situation easily corrected.

INAPPROPRIATE BEHAVIOR
No Other Word For It Than Taboo

There is one basic therapist-client rule: *you* do the touching, *they* do the receiving, and that is that! This subject entails the most complex circumstances of all those covered in this book.

One of my experiences in this category occurred with a male client while employed at a spa. I was working on a gentleman's quadriceps when he placed his hand on mine and pressed it harder into his leg. I didn't say anything but shook my hand loose (a *definite* "hint") and proceeded to continue the massage, whereupon he again placed his hand over mine and moved it toward his groin area. I released my hand again and had him turn over. Now ... I could have chosen to end this massage at that time, but made the decision to give him one more chance. There were no more attempts; however, even though he was one of the spa owner's best friends, I stipulated with the front desk that I would not work on him again. I realized he had been testing me for my level of interest in his advances, and wasn't planning on trying anything further after my responses–which was my purpose and very obvious reason in turning him over. Without having to speak a word, my message had been loud and clear. And the message to you is to *set your boundaries without any hesitation*!

And now we come to the subject that is totally and completely taboo from the perspective of female massage therapists: "grinding the table." Such an action is deliberate, suggestive, disrespectful, and grounds for ending the massage session immediately! Under *NO* circumstances should you continue! With a professional and firm manner, say, "This is inappropriate behavior that I am not comfortable with. The massage is over," and leave the room. I asked my manager to handle this client when he came out; he was not allowed to return. Male massage therapists may have a slightly different perspective, say a few words such as, "Not here, Buddy," or choose another appropriate course of action.

For these reasons, female massage therapists should seriously consider never giving a massage to a male stranger unless there are sufficient other people around, or at least one that you know and trust with your welfare. Likewise, male massage therapists need to consider the possibility of devious false accusations from female clients who are strangers. Should a female client attempt inappropriate comments or suggestive advances with male therapists, or clients of either gender toward a massage therapist of the same sex, the recommendation is the same.

In such situations it is up to you and your manager whether or not you would expect payment. In some instances it depends on when during the massage the event occurred. If it was in the first 15 minutes, I would suggest simply ending the massage and leaving it at that; if it was toward the end, I would suggest ending the massage but prorating the charge according to time.

Summary: Act professionally and most adults will respond accordingly. If they do not, then you not only have the *right*, you *should* end the massage at any inappropriate action and leave the room. Ultimately, what you may choose to do in any given situation will depend on your own levels of uneasiness, tolerance, intuition, and the circumstances. The key is to be prepared in your own mind concerning your boundaries and your reputation.

INTENTIONAL EXPOSURE
Not A Great Idea

There was an instance of this nature when I worked at a massage clinic and was scheduled to massage the husband of my boss. Having worked on him once before, when he arrived I led him back into the massage room, we exchanged the usual basic chit-chat, and I left so he could get ready. He was lying face down and every now and then would make a comment about this or that. At one point I turned my back to get some liniment just as he was asking me a question. I answered and turned around to witness him raising himself up onto his side–knowingly exposing the unclothed lower half of his body. He then questioned, "What was that? I didn't hear what you said."

That I was dealing with my boss's husband made this a bit more of a delicate situation in that moment. However, within nanoseconds my course of action came with great clarity! I stepped back to the table, answered him again, proceeded to gently but firmly push his body back down to the table, and started to work again. I continued the massage as though nothing had happened. After the massage was finished and he had left, I approached the manager and discussed this rather awkward subject, explaining I was uncomfortable working with him and would not do it again. When she then attempted to talk me into a change of mind, to just brush the situation aside, I realized that because he was the co-owner of the company his behavior was being excused. My decision remained the same.

Remember that if you are not comfortable, you will not be giving your best, *and* you would be sacrificing your own needs for others–something you do not want to do. *Do not jeopardize your integrity*. Stick with what your gut instinct is telling you. Intuition is your best friend in such situations.

MOANS AND GROANS
Oh Me, Oh My

Now *this* subject can sometimes make for a rather awkward situation–most especially so if there are other people in close hearing range of your room. What I am talking about here are the vocal sighs and sounds that escape when something really feels good. Many people express their feelings of relaxation and release of tension through sounds. There may be times when these releases are rather loud and might take you by surprise. The real difficulty comes when someone unintentionally sounds very sensuous with their relaxation releases!

One time I was working on another massage therapist after hours when we were the only ones in the establishment. She became very vocal, but I was able to make jokes about it with her because we were friends. Another time I felt quite uncomfortable with a client who was moaning and groaning, aware that anyone walking by really might be questioning what was happening behind my closed door, so in a gentle and polite voice I said, "I realize this must feel very good, but there are other clients and therapists that might be wondering what's going on back here." I was fortunate that she was able to laugh at herself, and quieted down a bit.

Such a situation is definitely one of the more awkward to bring up since the client's comfort level in all areas is to be considered first. Perhaps, with some, you might say, "I'm glad to know you are relaxing. Focus now on taking those feelings of relaxation deeper into your body and allowing them to be soothing." Use your discretion.

NUDITY AND SHENANIGANS
Just Keep Your Cool!

Walking in on someone naked … well, there *are* places in this world where nudity is common in the massage room, but if you've explained your rules, it should not be in *your* room!

Still in massage school, we had just begun giving massages to outside clients. This was to be my first male client (other than fellow students) and I naturally was a little apprehensive. Knocking on the door, I entered the room, looked toward the table, and noticed my client was lying on top of the sheets with nothing on. I immediately swiveled 180 degrees and was on my way out the door, saying, "Please lie *under* the sheet." He answered, "Oh, I'm too hot," to which I responded, "Then please cover up with the *towel*."

Regaining a measure of my composure, I returned to the room and went through the motions of a massage without being totally focused, to say nothing of my discomfort level. I had not been prepared for such blatant disrespect and inappropriate shenanigans.

What have I learned since then? Not to give my power away; that the massage therapist is the one in control in a massage room! A good response that does not give your client room for argument is, "Oops, I thought I had made myself clear. I prefer that you be covered during the massage. I'll just leave the room for a few seconds so you can get under the sheet," and walk out. Be confident and politely firm. If you act as though you were startled or affected in any way, the person will sense this and may continue to act out. Take a moment to take a few deep breaths before re-entering the room.

There is the possibility for an additional situation to occur, and this will take discernment on your part. We all know that touch can stimulate certain feelings. Some people are very aware of the difference between therapeutic touch and erotic touch. If, however, your client is not–which may happen on occasion with a client that has never had a massage before–there may be a reaction. This does not mean that the reaction was intentional or that your client was making advances. There have been times when I knew my client was completely embarrassed. In such a situation, I changed the pressure of my touch and continued with the massage. If either I or my client still seemed uncomfortable (you can determine this simply by "tuning in" to his energy), then I very casually had him turn over.

PULLING THE SHEET OR TOWEL OFF, OR TO ONE SIDE
Particularly In Slow Motion

This is *such* an unmistakably clear "Red Flag." Do *not* let any clients get away with it. Such an action is an obvious, albeit non-verbal, statement of intention.

A male client came in from out of town to the spa where I was working. He was from another state and said he received massage weekly. After giving my speech about what he should remove and where he should be on the table, I left the room. When I returned he was lying face up and was naked. I turned away and stated, "Sir, I need you under the sheet." He quickly let me know he never used a sheet because it was too hot for him. With my eyes averted, I handed him a towel and stated he needed to at least cover up with it. He argued. I insisted. He followed my instructions for about five minutes into the massage, whereupon he thought he would be clever and began *sssllllooowwwlly* moving the towel to one side … as if I wasn't going to notice! I moved the towel back. I was agitated and uncomfortable, and his behavior made it obvious he was not there to receive a therapeutic massage. Deciding not to waste any more time, I told him the massage was over, turned around, walked out, and went straight to the manager, who handled his departure.

Place a boundary and stick to it. Your personal integrity and reputation depend on it.

SECTION V

ACNE
Pesky Little Devils

Acne is a condition that can be either virtually unnoticeable or quite obvious. In fact, some people may not even know they have pores that are blocked, especially if they are not easily visible. Personally, I have always avoided severe acne–wherever it is. Should you ever need to explain why you are not including a specific area, simply say you "do not want to irritate the problem area." Never has anyone been upset when the explanation was given in those terms. But rarely will you find the client who wants you to touch their face if they have acne. You may, however, have a client who has back acne and not think twice about what you may encounter.

In my fledgling career I had been asked to massage a woman at her daughter's home. She did not speak very fluent English, so her daughter served as an interpreter during our initial chat time, explaining what her mother was experiencing, where she would like me to concentrate on her body, etc. I was massaging her back and was pressing firmly while moving my hands down to her waist–totally unsuspecting and unprepared for what happened next. A fountain of pus spurted upwards toward the ceiling. Surprised and shocked, at that precise moment I had no idea what, exactly, I was to do with the substance that now was lying on her back. I quickly became aware that my client was sleeping through this "ordeal" … how, I wasn't sure, but there she was, snoring peacefully.

What to do? Well, even though I was feeling a little panicked and somewhat nauseated, my automatic reaction was to grab some tissue while wondering what I might say to this dear woman if she wakened during this procedure. When the tissue wasn't enough to take care of my situation and I had also detected it had a specific odor, I scurried after more tissue and a towel with warm water and soap. I washed her back as gently as possible while she remained silent and sleeping–a gift in the midst of it all! The rest of her massage was with the lightest pressure I have ever used, *but* I had learned henceforth to avoid any area of thick, and therefore suspect, tissue.

My client lay asleep through the entire massage. Should any similar situation occur for you and your client happens to be awake and questions you about what you might be doing as you use a tissue or warm towel, act as normal as possible and respond with, "We just had a small outburst from a pore, but everything's fine. Just stay relaxed."

SKIN IRREGULARITIES
A Sensitive Subject

This can be a big concern for a massage therapist. When what we deal with *is* skin, and we have direct contact with whatever may be *on* the skin, then of course we are constantly aware of what may or may not be *happening* with one's skin. While some schools have specific classes dedicated to contagious diseases, others do not. And if you are not used to seeing or diagnosing skin disorders, you may have difficulty recognizing the difference between those that are contagious and those that are not. Plus, some clients may choose to tell you about a condition they are experiencing (maybe eczema or psoriasis) or they may leave it for you to notice and question. If you do not know what it is you are faced with, politely ask, "Please share with me the nature of your skin disorder" (or rash, or inflamed area, etc.). If you do not wish to ask, or the condition is contraindicated to massage, simply explain to your client that you are not going to massage over a particular area because you do not want it to become irritated.

One of my clients had come for a salt scrub followed by a massage. We met, went through the details, and I left the room for her to prepare. After I had been working on her extremities I undraped her tummy and found it was covered with scaly patches she had not mentioned. She immediately said, "They aren't contagious; it's psoriasis." Although I knew this to be true, because of the amount of patches, I was not comfortable working on the area. I explained that the combination of salt and scrubbing would irritate her condition and that I would work around it but wouldn't recommend working directly on it. She accepted this explanation.

If you are not comfortable touching a certain area of the body for whatever reason and do not have or wish to use the gloves that are made especially for massage therapists for this purpose, then do not. You will find it helpful to have appropriate comments to offer if any client asks why or counters your decision. Speak firmly and authoritatively, but politely.

SURGICAL MAKE-OVERS
Easy Does It!

Plastic surgery has become very popular and can be a very common situation to encounter on your massage table. Make it a part of your pre-massage chat to ask your clients if they have had any type of plastic surgery, especially within the past year. Some people are loathe to admit to certain procedures, but because you will likely be massaging the areas in question and need to know how long it has been since the surgery and if there were any complications, you might express to your clients that it is more beneficial for *them* if you have this information. And it certainly will put you more at ease. As with any surgery, a doctor's permission is a requirement before proceeding with massage–no matter what your client may tell you.

I have heard it all. One person called me for an appointment stating she had just received breast augmentation three days prior and that her back was in a lot of pain. She wanted me to come to her home right away. I asked her if she had clearance from her doctor to receive massage. "My doctor said it was fine," was her reply. I then asked her if she would mind *my* calling him just to make sure. "Oh, well, I'll call him" was her response. She did not call me again.

Under any and all circumstances, if a client is asking for massage and has had recent surgery, for your professional protection you need their doctor's permission in writing. It is as simple as that.

BOTOX

Many people do not think of Botox as a precaution they need to share when undergoing a pre-massage chat. Yet it is advised not to have any kind of pressure applied to the area during the first few days following an injection. Make sure they understand you are only asking to help keep them safe.

FACE LIFTS/OTHER FACIAL WORK

In my experience, most of the time people who have had any facial work done prefer not to have their faces touched, even long after they have healed. One of my clients, who had undergone a face lift several years prior and was completely healed, asked me to work on her face "gently."

BREAST AUGMENTATION

If my experiences in this category are any measure at all, you will undoubtedly have a number of clients who have had breast implant surgery. Depending on the size and how recent their procedure, it may be uncomfortable and/or impossible for them to lie prone. One suggestion is to roll some towels and place them above and below the breasts. Or you may want to try placing these clients on their sides, slightly leaning them into the table as long as they find this position comfortable. Ask if they have a preference about which position they think might be easier for them.

LIPOSUCTION

The procedure of any surgery can be the makings of a dangerous massage. Since every case is different and people respond differently to surgical procedures, please wait for a doctor's permission before performing any massage on someone that has received any surgery [see "Surgical Make-overs" above].

One female client came to me two days after tummy liposuction stating, "My belly is so hard and painful–will you please massage it?" The answer is NO! She stated her doctor had said it would be alright, and I still said no. There is too much at stake: *do not* put your career and your clients' health in danger by believing what everyone states. I politely told my client I simply was too uncomfortable with massaging her this soon after her surgery and had not been educated to massage after this type of surgery. Your client may be upset but, professionally speaking, there should be no other choice. Some offices employ massage therapists to work on clients directly after surgery. If you are not employed by the doctor that did the actual surgery, then, I feel, you must wait.

FEET AND TOES
Their Troubles And Woes

They carry us to and fro. More information below.

For FOOT ODOR, See BODY ODOR

CALLUSES
An All-Too-Common Foot Condition

Foot calluses can be caused by going barefoot a lot or by wearing shoes that fit your feet improperly. Having calluses usually should not interfere with massage technique unless the condition is exaggerated.

Several years practicing massage had indoctrinated me well with what I would call "unpleasantries," but one day a client came to my table who has become memorable among my experiences in this category. She wanted to relax and gave me no other comments or instructions. As I was working on the backs of her legs, I noticed the soles of her feet were completely covered with about an inch of thick calluses. Not only was the entire area hard, it was black and looked incapable of being scrubbed clean. Large cracks went deep into her heels. It was difficult for me to understand how she even could walk, or how her shoes possibly could fit. Nor could I comprehend why anyone would allow such a condition to occur without seeking help.

Obviously such a condition falls outside the realm of massage therapy. I made no mention of it and simply avoided the area below her ankles. Should she have made a comment about her feet, I was prepared to be honest, suggesting the area looked impossible to penetrate with massage and perhaps she might consider seeing a podiatrist to have the calluses removed, and then make another appointment to have her feet worked on. As with all other situations, such comments are to be presented politely and professionally.

TOE FUNGUS/ATHLETE'S FOOT
Another Foot Wonder

Putting aside the fact of amazement that so many people do *not* have a problem presenting others with such an unpleasant situation to work with, because fungus *can* be contagious, it is a subject you *must* discuss with your client. Questions should include whether or not they are aware that what they have is, indeed, a fungus; have they seen a doctor about their condition; were they told their condition was contagious (some fungi are, some are not); were they given any medication or ointment to help control or cure the fungus; if appearing on their feet, has the fungus ever been on their fingers (and vice versa); are they aware if the fungus may have spread to any other area on their body. Should any of your clients indicate they had *not* seen a doctor about their condition, you might explain that it can be a serious situation because it may continue to spread, that there are effective treatments for their condition, and they may wish to see a dermatologist or podiatrist as soon as possible.

There are various images of fungus to which you may be exposed. I have seen toes with a small area affected; entire toes and surrounding skin covered in fungus; toes with nails that were barely hanging on because the fungus had eaten away any healthy tissue; toes with no nails at all; skin that was so cracked and brittle from fungus that I knew it must have been active for years.

Understand that you have absolutely no obligation to include fungus-infected areas in your massage. In a professional attitude and manner, tell any clients with this condition that you will not be able to massage the infected areas but will spend extra time on another part of the body instead, and ask if there is an area of preference.

THE HUMAN PLUMBING
SYSTEM
When The Call Comes, Listen Up

How you present the delicate subject of having to use the "facilities" can put your clients at ease about this normal, necessary, and healthy function of our human bodies. Sharing the location of the Rest Room in your pre-massage chat is a subtle way of offering your clients that option before they get on the table. Inform them that particularly when massaging the abdomen, the bladder and intestines have a way of getting "stirred up", and they should feel comfortable in interrupting the massage at any time if they wish to use the Rest Room. Your clients will not only appreciate this information, they may be more able to fully relax during the massage without a worrisome "What if?"

I gave a massage to a woman that I had made sure knew where the ladies room was prior to beginning the hour. It was a relaxing time–nothing out of the ordinary–so I thought. Unfortunately, as soon as I finished she jumped up saying "I've had to use the bathroom for a half hour." I felt terrible–not because it was my fault, but because I knew she hadn't been able to really relax.

The same applies to the massage therapist! Should you need to excuse yourself, whisper to your client that you need to leave, to take a few deep breaths and stay relaxed, and you will return in a few minutes.

It will be a big deal only if you allow it to be.

SECTION VI

THE PERFECT ATMOSPHERE
Importantè!

You want to be particular about the environment your clients enter when they arrive for a massage. Make sure the surrounding areas are clean and organized. This includes the bathroom your clients will be using, the lobby, and any other areas they will see. If you are in a space where clients may be waiting while you finish with another client or are preparing the room for them, it's always a nice touch to provide pleasant magazines and articles, including books or brochures about the benefits of massage therapy and other related subjects. This will serve as a calming agent as they shift from their hurried world to a relaxing massage.

The first thing clients notice when entering a massage room is the type of lighting and the temperature; adjust these according to your clients' needs and the type of massage you're giving (i.e., a relaxation massage in a spa environment vs. a sports massage for a 250 lb. athlete). Think ahead and prepare the room to exude relaxation: music playing softly; a soft glow from lighted candles or a low-wattage lamp; the gentle scent of a pleasant essential oil. Everything around them must whisper "*peaceful environment.*" For some, receiving massage is a rare occurrence; for others, a desperate escape from the stresses of everyday life. They should begin to feel relaxed the *instant* they step through the doorway. You will want to have a specified place in your room where your clients can hang their clothing, and also a chair/seat where they can easily take off and put on their shoes.

You want your table to be an experience unto itself. The appeal of your massage table can be cozy and inviting or cold and un-welcoming. Everything about it should express that you care about your client's comfort. Even if you have a padded table, ALWAYS use some sort of thick padding such as an egg-crate cushion, a fleece pad, or foam to allow a soft barrier between the sheet and the table. (I chose to use a fleece pad and was told on numerous occasions that it made all the difference in the world–plus, they're machine washable!) My personal experiences on tables without any padding were cold and uninviting!

Using good quality, clean sheets (twin bed size works perfectly) is very important. This is an absolute must for any massage environment! Using a clean set of sheets for each client goes without saying, so have at least enough sheets for any one-day's use–plus one spare just in case something happens. There are detergents that specifically target oil stains on sheets, but if they become permanently stained or worn out from use/washing many times, it's time for a new set. People will definitely be turned off by the sight of stains and/or frayed edges.

Have a few blankets on hand. During massage some people get chilly and others can become too warm, so lightweight cotton blankets are usually recommended. It is easier to adjust the comfort level for your client without hindering your work by having to maneuver a large, thick blanket.

Be conscious of the head rest ... not only the cover (which, in my opinion, should be soft and flexible), but also the position of your client's head while on the head rest. It is up to *you* to determine where each person's head should be; every body is different, and different angles can be more comfortable for one than for another. I recommend tables with adjustable head rests for this specific reason. While this is taught in massage schools, it is surprising how many therapists forget to check or ask if their clients' necks are comfortable. More times than not, clients will simply forego mentioning their discomfort rather than speaking up–it is your job to notice and make the appropriate adjustment.

Any bolsters or pillows you use should be covered in soft, washable material and not be stuffed too thick. Some people may enjoy a hot water bottle wrapped in a thin towel at their feet.

Take the time to "test drive" your table. Lie on it to get a "bird's eye view" of what your clients will be seeing as they look above and below the table and around the room. Having received many massages as well as given them, as a client I observed what felt good, what was working, and what wasn't. It can be a beneficial practice for you to pay attention while you're on the receiving end and incorporate any insights that may enhance your own massage techniques. For example, as I was lying on my back during one of my "receiving" massages, I glanced at the ceiling and saw dead flies and insects in the fluorescent light; this was not a pleasant sight and did not create the cozy environment I was looking to experience.

The message is: *All these things make a difference*!!

MASSAGE THERAPY JOB OPPORTUNITIES

Fortunately, the popularity of massage therapy is continuously growing. There is an ever-increasing range of opportunities for therapists in many different areas of service as awareness of the many healing benefits massage offers becomes more prevalent. You may find yourself wondering where it is you would fit in as a working therapist. When considering the type of environment that would best suit your personality and circumstances, think about your lifestyle: what schedule you would like to keep, how many hours you are willing to work, what type of therapy you prefer. Consider how much interaction you would like to have with your clients, whether or not you are a "people person," are looking to pamper people, or are driven by challenges. Ask yourself what attracted you to the field of massage therapy, and why.

Establishing your own private practice is a popular first choice even though it takes time to build up regular, loyal clients. Many therapists choose to begin their massage careers by scheduling massages in the evenings and on weekends until their clientele is sufficient for them to leave their full-time job. Others prefer this arrangement as a permanent second income.

Salons and spas are generally the places most commonly associated with massage availability. Those who frequent establishments of this nature are more inclined toward receiving relaxation massage.

Sports massage is a huge business opportunity. Many sports teams and professional athletes–including the Olympics–employ massage therapists that travel with them as part of their support staff.

Massage Clinics are a popular choice for people searching for massage. Usually this type of place has a number of therapists offering a full spectrum of different massage techniques; a known environment for regular clientele.

Businesses are recognizing the benefits of massage for their employees. There were a number of times I was called into a corporate environment for chair massage work, giving 10- to 15-minute mini-massages. This is very rewarding work; people who sit at desks all day need not only the physical relaxation but the mental distraction for greater stress relief, and are usually pleasantly surprised at how invigorating a short massage can be without having to remove any clothing. Often you will receive a number of clients from this type of marketing.

Massage therapy is expanding to more and more doctors' offices. Many chiropractors and osteopaths are incorporating massage into their practices. It is always a plus to be on a doctor's referral list. I even have had my personal business cards posted in a dentist/orthodontist's office. (It never hurts to ask!)

Some hospitals and medical doctors are acknowledging the benefits of including massage therapy among their treatment modalities. Medical massage can be very fulfilling to the therapists who feel they would like to reach out to those dealing with physical challenges. There are some hospitals that are incorporating alternative healing modalities in their facilities.

Some Plastic Surgeons are finding the benefits of including massage therapy in their offices to help with post-op recovery.

Even the older generations are receiving help from treatments that include touch therapy.

If you're interested in traveling and want the security of a steady income and clientele right away, you may want to consider working on a cruise ship or at a resort. Down time can be spent in different ports discovering different towns or on the beach catching some fun in the sun.

Many high-class hotels offer on-site spas. Since there are a number of people that include massage as a "must have" during a vacation or while traveling, hotels can be good places to put out cards, be an on-call therapist, or be employed full- or part-time.

There is no limit to those you can serve as a massage therapist. Finding your own niche and what brings you joy can be a fun opportunity to explore all kinds of work environments. New and amazing opportunities are being expanded all the time to include this wonderful healing modality. If you feel massage would benefit a certain type of individual not yet being reached, then, by all means, reach out and take it on!

HELPFUL HINTS

- Allow yourself enough time before your client arrives (or before you leave home) to make sure you have everything you need.

- If you share a table with another therapist, don't forget to check its height when setting up.

- Choose comfortable but presentable clothing suitable to your working environment. Nothing too tight and nothing too loose. And always wear very comfy but supportive shoes—your feet and back will thank you!

- If only fluorescent lighting is available, don't turn it on. Buy a lamp and use soft lighting.

- Adjust the room temperature at a level that is comfortable for your clients. Take into consideration the time of year, and remember they're the ones with their clothes off!

- Something I used and heard repeatedly was a "favorite touch": having a hot water bottle or a hot pack to place under my clients' feet. They seemed to fully enjoy this small luxury!

- Using an exercise ball for seated work at your table is a great way to save your back. It's comfortable and glides easily without noise.

- Always make sure you have plenty of oil and/or lotion for the day. You never know when someone will need more, depending on skin type. Consider using liniment; keep two kinds on hand in case of sensitivities, and always remember to ask your clients if they have allergies to certain products.

- This isn't a "must," but it's always a nice touch to warm your oil or lotion. There are warmers you can buy that the bottles sit in so they are always at the right temperature for use.

- Do all you can to warm your hands before you touch the body. Wash them in warm water and/or rub them together to get the circulation moving. If they still seem to be on the chilly side and you need to begin the massage, warn your client that your hands will warm up within a few minutes.

- I recommend you do not touch your face or any other part of your body during massages. Keep a small towel within your reach. If you have an itch, you can easily rub the towel over the area without touching your skin with oily or greasy hands that have been touching another's body.

- Wash your hands thoroughly up to your elbows after each massage. Make sure to scrub off any residue of oil or lotion.

- Clean your bottles and containers often to avoid bacteria buildup.

- Keep nail clippers and files at work. Nails that are too long or broken will jab or scratch your clients and will inhibit the type of work you can do. Remove any dirt from under your nails. If you wear nail polish, you will make a better impression if it is not peeling.

- Schedule enough time between clients to change sheets, use the bathroom, and sip some water. Some working environments will make your appointments back to back; this may work for a few sessions, but you'll soon realize squeezing everything needed into a few minutes and then calming yourself to appear the peaceful massage therapist can become rather hectic.

Always take breaks during your work days, especially for lunch and/or dinner.
Allow additional breaks in a heavily scheduled period for clients who are late or other interruptions.

- Generally speaking, most people relax quicker with soft, gentle music in the background. Have a few selections to interchange. Make sure you can turn the music up, down, or off if your clients prefer silence or simply do not enjoy the specific music that is playing.
Always listen to any new music before using it during a massage to make sure it is suitable for massage throughout its entirety.

- Have a small assortment of hair combs, clips, and barrettes in your room for use in keeping your clients' hair from interfering with your massage and to keep it tidy and free from oil/lotion.

- Place a small dish close to where your clients disrobe. This will save the inevitable phone calls later stating, "I forgot my earrings" or, "Have you found my gold necklace?" They can place their jewelry in the dish and have it all together when it is time to leave.

- Do everything you can to make your clients' time with you memorable in a positive way.

- I've had many highly trained therapists "plow" into me, which was far from relaxing. My suggestion is to ease your way into that first touch and finish with a gentle release as well. Even the deepest massage should begin and end with ease. This way you won't startle your client or leave them feeling like they've just been put "through the wringer."

- Traveling with your table? If this answer is "yes", then my advice is to invest in a carrying cart; it's well worth every penny. Tables aren't always heavy, but they can be awkward. Save your back lots of undue physical stress.

• Always be prepared! A great idea to form as a habit is keeping a bag filled with what you will need at work or while giving a massage in another establishment, ready to pick up and go. This will save you those times of realizing too late that you've forgotten something you needed!

• Once you've finished the therapy, never leave your client to fend for themselves; provide closure. Ask them if they have any questions and tell them what you found. Suggest stretching, and depending on where they may have specific issues, you may want to recommend certain stretching exercises for the most common "problem" areas (i.e., neck, low back, calves, etc.). Educate yourself on different stretches. It's helpful to keep a book on hand for reference and to show clients, if needed. There are many reputable choices on the market. Always mention the benefits of drinking water after receiving massage.

• Have fun with your clients!

• Take care of YOURSELF! As massage therapists, we have the tendency not to practice what we preach. Take the time to *receive* massage–especially in your shoulders, arms, wrists, hands, fingers, and back. These areas can take a beating, so be especially conscious about their care and you will have a greater chance of extending the life of your career.

978-0-595-45134-0
0-595-45134-9

Printed in the United States
110449LV00003B/146/A